" *Firstly may I say what a user friendly book this is. The idea of stretching in the horizontal plane has been my philosophy for a considerable length of time. As an osteopath I have taught a stretch class to patients for the last twenty years, most of whom have learned how to look after their own musculoskeletal system and no longer need or seek treatment. I can thoroughly recommend this book with its common-sense approach to exercise.* "

SHEILA LEE
REGISTERED OSTEOPATH – CLINICAL ERGONOMIST, LONDON, UK

" *Your book is outstanding. I think you came up with something which is quite unique.* "

DR HARRY WALLACE
PROFESSOR AT PALMER COLLEGE OF CHIROPRACTIC, USA

" *Treating your back is like dental brushing for an hour is not good enoug.., ... day for a couple of minutes. This is why I strongly recommend this book with daily exercise for a more healthy back.* "

MARK VAN STRATEN
NIKE'S EUROPEAN PHYSIOTHERAPIST

" *The exercises are very easy to follow and an excellent idea. The exercises are standard back exercises that we give to people with back problems. I like the way this book encourages people to take responsibility for the care of their back. The general principles in this book seem to fit with many of the current theories about how to treat mechanical back pain.* "

DR DEBORAH SKEIL
SPINAL REHABILITATION CONSULTANT, DEPARTMENT OF PHYSICAL MEDICINE AND
REHABILITATION, CHRISTIAN MEDICAL COLLEGE AND HOSPITAL, VELLORE, INDIA

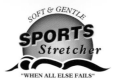

SOFT & GENTLE
SPORTS *Stretcher*
"WHEN ALL ELSE FAILS"

At last a "Sports" Stretcher for the fit & healthy

The difference between the *'Soft & Gentle'* Backstretcher and the larger 'Sports' version is that the *'Soft & Gentle'* Backstretcher was designed to help individuals with back problems. If a person is in pain or has anything wrong with their back then the product to choose is the award winning *'Soft & Gentle'* Backstretcher. Healthy individuals with no history of backache can use the Sports version to increase suppleness. Athletes use it to increase their flexibility. Gymnastic individuals or people familiar with exercising and who are still 'working out' use it as the ultimate in "warm up" or "cool down" stretching. You do not need to be a large or tall person to use the larger Sports version, but you do need a greater degree of flexibility in the spine. If you are a stiff or inflexible individual by nature then the *'Soft & Gentle'* Backstretcher is the version for you. If your gym does not have a "Sports" stretcher, here's your chance to get your own!

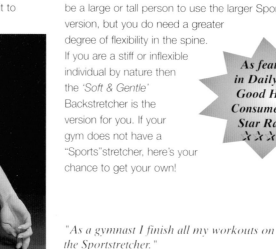

As featured in Daily Mail Good Health Consumer Test. Star Rating: ✗✗✗✗✗

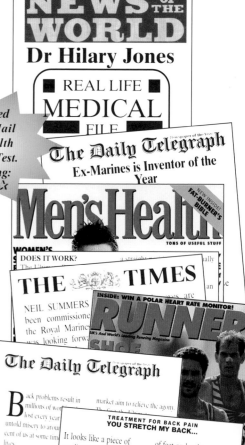

NEWS OF THE WORLD
Dr Hilary Jones
REAL LIFE MEDICAL FILE

The Daily Telegraph
Ex-Marines is Inventor of the Year

Men's Health

THE TIMES
NEIL SUMMERS been commissione the Royal Marines was looking forw

The Daily Telegraph

TREATMENT FOR BACK PAIN
YOU STRETCH MY BACK...
It looks like a piece of medieval torture equipment. In fact, it is quite the opposite. Far from inflicting pain, the Backstretcher provides a surprisingly comfortable way of alleviating it.

"As a gymnast I finish all my workouts on the Sportstretcher."
FIONA, 33, MOTHER OF TWO, SURREY.

Product	Price Each
SOFT & GENTLE NECKstretcher	£29.95
SOFT & GENTLE BACKstretcher	£79.00
SOFT & GENTLE "Sports"stretcher	£99.00

YOUR GUARANTEE: Order without risk. If for any reason you are not satisfied with your order from us, just return it to us within 30 days for an immediate replacement or a full refund.

ORDERING HAS NEVER BEEN EASIER...
☎ **0700 222 5724** VISA MasterCard

OR Simply send, together with your payment, to:
**ENANEF Limited,
Beechwood House, King George's Hill, Abinger Bottom,
Dorking, Surrey RH5 6JW.**

" *Since I've been using your back exercises/routine I can keep my schedule without the twinges in my back as I move through my busy day as a doctor. Being pain free through the day is a wonderful gift. Even doctors need to look after themselves. I can think of no better way than using your routine.*
Thank you, Neil. "

DR SHEILA PHILLIPS
SANTA MONICA, CALIFORNIA, USA

" *The book is very impressive. As an exercise physiologist working with elite sportsmen and women I will be only too happy to recommend this excellently compiled book to them. A few minutes a day spent on exercising your back in the correct way is time well spent both for the present and future well-being.* "

DR PAUL BALSOM
EXERCISE PHYSIOLOGIST, SWEDISH NATIONAL FOOTBALL TEAM, STOCKHOLM, SWEDEN

" *Excellent, clear photographs throughout the book. The structure for each exercise is very clear and very precise. By sub-dividing each exercise into starting position, movement and effect this allows the mechanics of the movement to be explained. However, even more significantly for a text of this type, it provides the reader with a rationale as to why the movement is being performed. This is very rare for a text of this type. With an ever increasing older population, I was delighted to see that this population was catered for in this book. Overall, I would highly recommend this text for individuals of all ages and fitness levels.* "

VISH UNNITHAN PH.D.
PROFESSOR OF EXERCISE & SPORT SCIENCE, UNIVERSITY OF SAN FRANCISCO, USA

The Soft & Gentle Neckstretcher is designed to cradle the neck along the base of the skull, keeping the head and spinal column in the correct alignment.

Made of wood and shaped in the reverse image of the curvature of the neck. A channel in the centre prevents the bones at the top of the spine rubbing against the wood.

Thumb-like nodules apply pressure to the muscles and acupressure points on either side of the spine. To use it, lie on the floor, and rest the neck and head back over the Neckstretcher.

The weight of the head gives gentle traction to the neck, while the nodules have a massaging effect, designed to relieve muscular aches and tension.

The Neckstretcher was invented by British exercise physiologist Neil Summers. Its forerunner, the Backstretcher, won the Invention Of The Year Award in 1995.

Mr Summers states 'Many people feel tension in the neck and shoulders, that doesn't drive them to visit the doctor, but if it

- *Comfortable and yet effective in releasing muscle tension*

- *Fully supports the neck*

- *Stable and made to last*

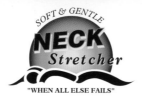

...The comfortable way to lose that neck pain!

causes a headache, they will usually take something to relieve the pain.'

'The Neckstretcher is an alternative. It helps with headaches. The secret is to use it little and often.'

Mr Summers says the Neckstretcher fights all neck tension-related conditions, including computer fatigue. A welcome side-effect is that by improving spinal alignment, posture is improved, which means people are less likely to suffer such conditions.

Most people in sedentary occupations will experience tension in the upper shoulders. This is often exacerbated by bad posture, particularly for those at desk-bound jobs or those who spend many hours driving.

Most of us tend to slouch, curving the spine and the shoulders forward. The more stressed we feel, the more we compress our necks and hunch our shoulders. Ideally, we should have the tension massaged out of our shoulders every hour or so.

The Neckstretcher works like a personal masseur, but has the added benefit of retraining the muscles.

Chiropractor Harry Wallace is researching pain, and is conducting trials into the Neck stretcher at the University of Iowa in America.

'Lying down is the optimum position for relieving inter-discal pressure, but we don't have any traction on the spine simply by being horizontal, which is what this device does,' says Dr Wallace.

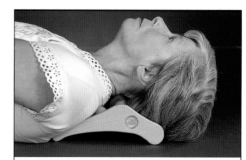

"Within minutes my neck pain had disappeared. I used to suffer with headaches and bad neck pain but now find the Neckstretcher invaluable in relieving my headaches."
DORIS. 62. RETIRED. YORKSHIRE.

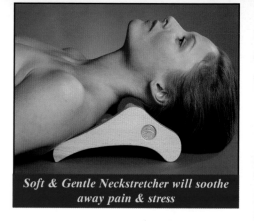

Soft & Gentle Neckstretcher will soothe away pain & stress

"It distracts the head and neck region without extension, which is the best way to use traction.

What interests me is the projections which push into the belly of the muscles in the neck and upper shoulders while they are being stretched by the traction.

When I do hands-on therapy, I manipulate the muscles, but they contract back afterwards

The Neckstretcher appears to have what we call the retainer effect. When an ortho-dontist puts a retainer (or brace) on the teeth, he is applying continuous traction on the jaw muscles, preventing them from contracting. The projections work in a similar way.

By pressing on the muscles while they are stretched, they interrupt the spring-back effect. In time, the muscles may be retrained into maintaining this position, as the jaw muscles are retrained by the retainer.

I have always used the Neckstretcher as a preventative tool for my headaches and it certainly has extraordinary capabilities," states Dr Wallace.

If Not 100% Satisfied Simply Return For A Full Refund

About the author

Neil Summers was an international lecturer in Physical Education. He formerly served with the British Royal Marine Special Forces, and has a Masters Degree from Springfield College, Mass, USA.

He now works as an exercise physiologist, advising major international corporations exactly how to design products for a healthy life. One of Neil's more famous inventions is the Ultimate Backstretcher, which was selected as British Invention of the Year, making Neil the British Inventor of the Year 1995.

As a Body Coach he has helped national heads of state, politicians, sports stars and a host of American, Japanese and European celebrities.

THE ART OF BACKSTRETCHING

NEIL SUMMERS

with

SHARRON DAVIES MBE

EnanefPress

"THOUSANDS OF PEOPLE AROUND THE WORLD HAVE ALREADY DISCOVERED HOW TO BEAT BACK PAIN"
with Neil Summers's – Backstretchers

At last ...
A Soft & Gentle Backstretcher
Beat back pain with added comfort

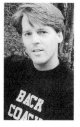

Neil Summers, award winning back coach and exercise physiologist, reviews the *Soft & Gentle* Backstretcher and explains how it has transformed his life.

Forced to leave the Royal Marines as a result of a serious and debilitating back problem, he now leads a fully active life and has never felt or looked better thanks to the *Soft & Gentle* Backstretcher.

"I had always led a very active life. I was diagnosed as suffering a debilitating back problem. The constant nagging aches became so painful I couldn't even sleep, let alone exercise.

I was discharged from the Royal Marines and urgently set about looking for some "miracle cure" to the back pain that ended my career so prematurely and was turning me into an invalid.

I refused to accept that nothing could be done and after months of reading everything I could on the subject I learnt that whilst there are many different causes, experts agreed that simply stretching the spine could relieve even

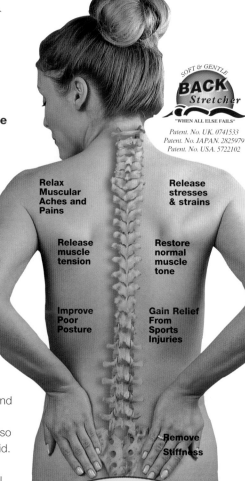

Relax Muscular Aches and Pains

Release stresses & strains

Release muscle tension

Restore normal muscle tone

Improve Poor Posture

Gain Relief From Sports Injuries

Remove Stiffness

30 DAY MONEY BACK GUARANTEE

SOFT & GENTLE
BACK Stretcher
"WHEN ALL ELSE FAILS"

Patent. No. UK. 0741533
Patent. No. JAPAN. 2825979
Patent. No. USA. 5722102

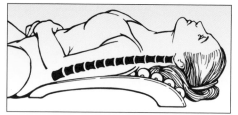

This natural stretch removes pressure from the discs by providing a mild form of traction

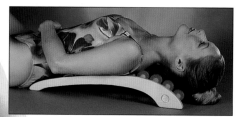

Lie back, relax and let gravity do the rest. The cushioned pads make this experience comfortable.

the most chronic back pain.

This was the clue I had been looking for. I set about designing a product that would enable anyone of any age to stretch their spine by simply lying down and relaxing. The result was the Soft & Gentle Backstretcher you see today.

Like all great ideas it is remarkably simple. It has won awards for The Great British Invention of the Year and The Best New Healthcare and Medical Product but most importantly it has helped thousands of people around the world treat and end their own back pain."

"to my surprise and delight, long term neck and shoulder pain faded away with my use of the back stretcher. In my opinion, this device has more potential than any other of its kind to reduce pain and suffering in back care today."
Dr Harry Wallace
Professor. Palmer College. Iowa, USA
(A leading authority in Chiropractic)

"for people who have back pain, poor posture, muscle spasm and restricted movement.... Safe, easy to use and effective in reducing tension and improving posture.... be of great help to many people who have back pain."
'Therapy Weekly'

"simple, effective and designed to meet a genuine need..."
'Hospital Doctor' the leading newspaper for medical professionals

Provides long lasting pain relief for back pain associated with:
- **ARTHRITIS**
- **STIFFNESS**
- **MUSCULAR ACHES & PAINS**
- **POOR POSTURE**
- **SPORTS INJURIES**

Try It In The Comfort Of Your Own Home

To Fiona and our three beautiful girls
Francesca, Georgina and Charlotte
in the hope that you are always blessed
with health, love and happiness

———————————

First published in Great Britain in 2000 by
Enanef Press
Beechwood House
King George's Hill
Dorking RH5 6JW
Tel: 0700 222 5724

A CIP catalogue record for this book
is available from the British Library

ISBN 0-9538123-0-8

Produced by Lennard Books
Editor: Michael Leitch
Design: Paul Cooper Design
Photography: William Taylor
Printed and bound in Singapore by Tien Wah Press

The Back Coach's
Equipment Guide

Contents

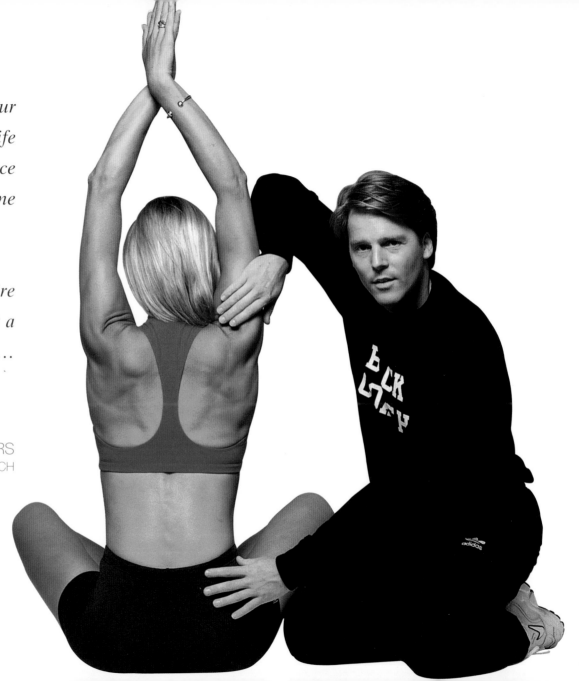

A healthy back is vital for our comfort and mobility throughout life but since we are all likely to experience some form of back pain at some time we must take precautions.

My philosophy applies whether you're a mum, an athlete, a celebrity or just a bad-back sufferer. My best advice is … stretch yourself!

NEIL SUMMERS
THE BACK COACH

Foreword

We are proud owners of a single spine and it will have to serve us a whole lifetime. But we do not take very good care of this precious and unique device! It is estimated that more than 80% of the population will suffer from back pain. But, strikingly, in about 90% of those cases a precise cause of the suffering will not be found despite all the investigative processes of modern medicine. Most problems are functional problems. There is nothing wrong with the back, it is just being misused. The back needs to move. The loads on the discs need to be relieved and the back muscles need to relax.

Neil Summers has brought together in this book a number of simple exercises which will help you achieve those goals. The book is easy to read and easy to use. A few minutes of care for your back every day will ensure a friendlier relationship with your spine!

I recommend this book not only to back sufferers but also as a preventative tool to all those who want to keep their back in shape.

DR MAREK SZPALSKI

Consultant in Orthopedic Surgery

Associate Professor, Free University of Brussels, Belgium

Adjunct Assistant Professor, Vanderbilt University, Nashville, USA

Senior Scientist, Hospital for Joint Diseases, New York University, USA

Co-editor of *Lumbar Segmental Instability* (Lippincott, 1998)

Final word

Low back pain remains a problem for many of us. In fact, about 75% of us will have a significant episode at some time in our life.

Neil Summers has developed a series of exercises which have some support in laboratory studies that we have conducted.

The book is beautifully illustrated and easy to follow. It is recommended to the chronic low back sufferer who has no serious medical conditions – this represents most people with lower back pain!

MALCOLM POPE DrMedSc, PhD

Professor and Chair of Health and Safety, Department of BioMedical

Physics and Director of the Liberty Centre, University of Aberdeen

Adjunct Professor, University of Patras, Greece

Adjunct Professor, University of Iowa, USA

Introduction

You will not find a more superb piece of machinery than your body. Unfortunately, it is seldom allowed to function in the way for which it was designed. The result, for the majority of us, is that we are rarely free from pain.

We constantly overload the back with tasks and habits that lead to poor posture. As we age, our back bends forwards and shortens and we lose the all-round flexibility that we had in our youth.

Most of our adult days are spent flexed forward, crumpled in a forward bending position, hunched over our everyday tasks. So insidious is this forward 'pull' of the head that we do not even notice it is happening. What makes things worse is that most of us have stopped using our bodies to move in any dynamic or athletic way at all. But if we do not let our back perform the varied array of movements it is capable of, we condemn ourselves to a life of aches and pains.

So, what can you DO about YOUR back?

Feedback

When you complete the full routine for a week - congratulate yourself. Well done! Did you notice how some of the exercises toward the end of the week were a little more demanding than the earlier ones? That's right. They are graded so that your back can become progressively stronger and able to carry out the more demanding routines.

So, now it is the end of the week. Even after just one week, you should be feeling the benefits of our backstretching routine.

All horizontal stretching opens out your back, easing out that hunched posture and giving your spine the chance to function as nature intended.

Sometimes it can take a little time to dissolve all the stiffness which has been building up over the years. Just be patient, and the results will come.

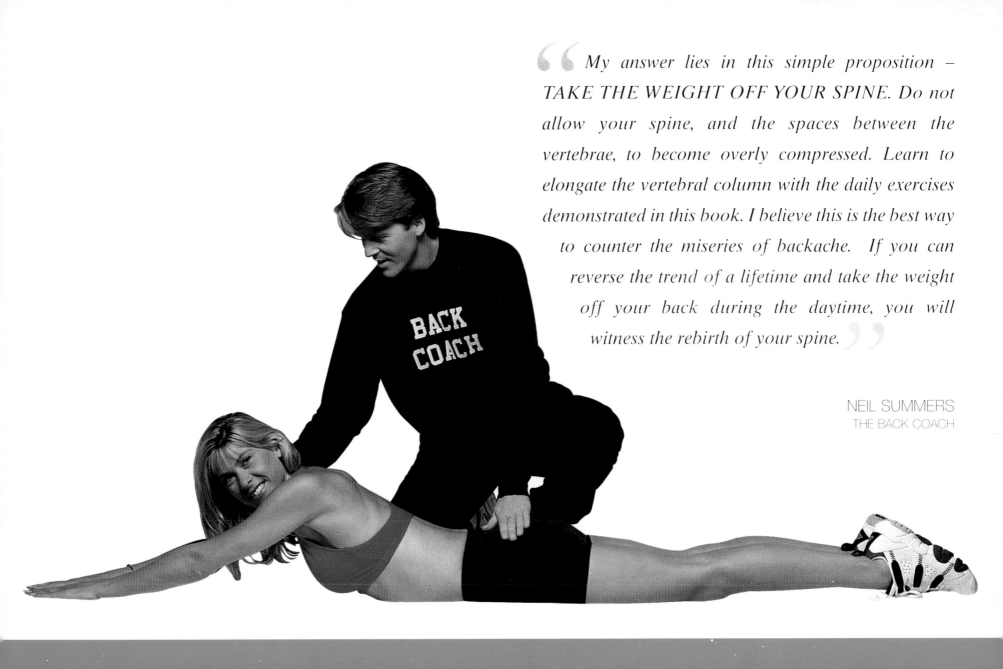

> " *My answer lies in this simple proposition –* **TAKE THE WEIGHT OFF YOUR SPINE.** *Do not allow your spine, and the spaces between the vertebrae, to become overly compressed. Learn to elongate the vertebral column with the daily exercises demonstrated in this book. I believe this is the best way to counter the miseries of backache. If you can reverse the trend of a lifetime and take the weight off your back during the daytime, you will witness the rebirth of your spine.* "

NEIL SUMMERS
THE BACK COACH

Cat on All-fours: Curl, Stretch and Walk

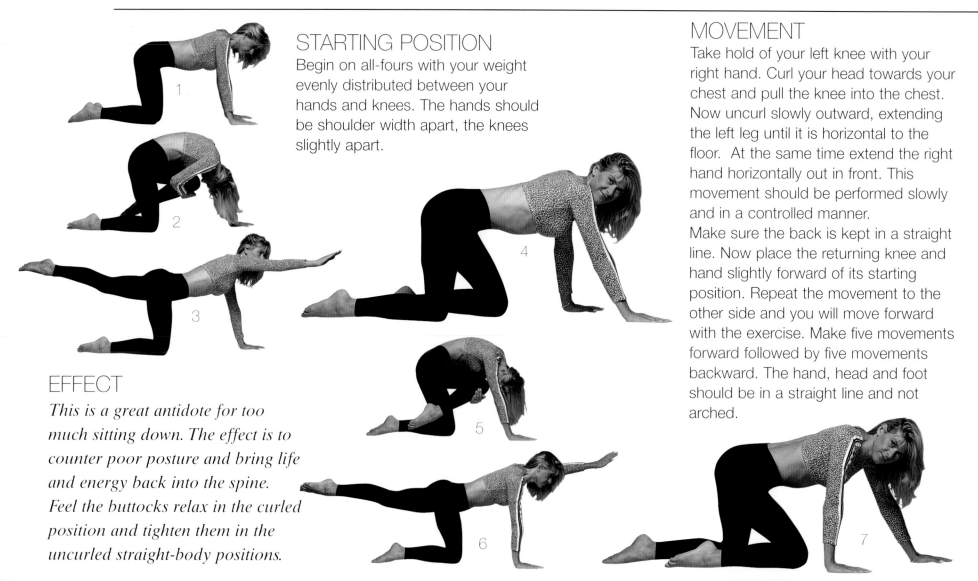

STARTING POSITION

Begin on all-fours with your weight evenly distributed between your hands and knees. The hands should be shoulder width apart, the knees slightly apart.

EFFECT

This is a great antidote for too much sitting down. The effect is to counter poor posture and bring life and energy back into the spine. Feel the buttocks relax in the curled position and tighten them in the uncurled straight-body positions.

MOVEMENT

Take hold of your left knee with your right hand. Curl your head towards your chest and pull the knee into the chest. Now uncurl slowly outward, extending the left leg until it is horizontal to the floor. At the same time extend the right hand horizontally out in front. This movement should be performed slowly and in a controlled manner.

Make sure the back is kept in a straight line. Now place the returning knee and hand slightly forward of its starting position. Repeat the movement to the other side and you will move forward with the exercise. Make five movements forward followed by five movements backward. The hand, head and foot should be in a straight line and not arched.

Backstretching
– to relieve backache

The good news, we are told, is that exercise is once more in fashion for the treatment of backache. However, this is only partly a good thing. In fact, not all exercise is good for the back - and certain forms of exercise are actually bad for it. That is why so many people merely make their back problems worse by exercising in the wrong way, and this in turn helps to perpetuate the myth that once you have a bad back, you will always have one. It does not need to be this way. By exercising in the correct way, stretching and strengthening your back, your aches and pains will be significantly diminished, resulting in a back that functions as it should … pain free.

As a remedy for back sufferers, bed-rest has been the most trusted friend of doctors through the centuries. However, we must realize why this should be so. In terms of body positioning, it is the act of going horizontal which helps us. By taking up this position, as we do each time we go to bed, we immediately remove the stresses and strains on the spine caused by the compressional effects of gravity. Literally, we take the weight off the spaces between the vertebrae. This is heaven to the damaged joint. It arrests further damage and allows the joint time to recover, repair and recuperate.

The whole story of the human back is very simple really. The back wants to move as it was designed to move. It yearns to be free to move again - fully elongated lengthways. You only have to look at our friends in the animal kingdom. Animals naturally open out their bodies when they move, and in the process reap the benefits of fully extended stretching, as opposed to the compressive forward-bending kind of movements that we are constantly making.

Both Knees Press against Chest - Rock

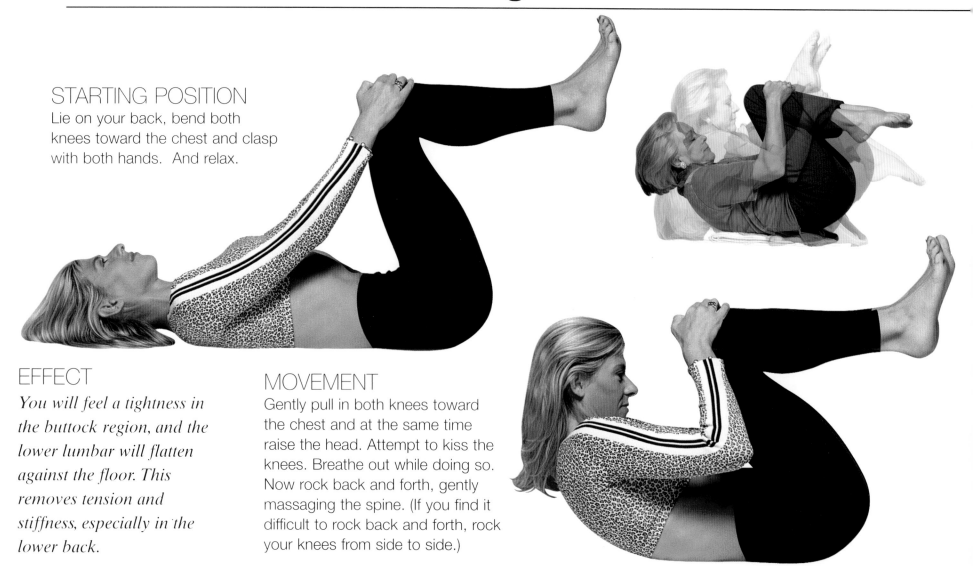

STARTING POSITION
Lie on your back, bend both knees toward the chest and clasp with both hands. And relax.

EFFECT
You will feel a tightness in the buttock region, and the lower lumbar will flatten against the floor. This removes tension and stiffness, especially in the lower back.

MOVEMENT
Gently pull in both knees toward the chest and at the same time raise the head. Attempt to kiss the knees. Breathe out while doing so. Now rock back and forth, gently massaging the spine. (If you find it difficult to rock back and forth, rock your knees from side to side.)

Backstretching
– to reduce back pain

Damage to the joints can occur in all kinds of ways - through sporting injuries, car accidents, hereditary complaints, through wear and tear or even the slightest of sudden awkward movements. Once damaged, the joints in the spine suffer a constant and never-ending downward pressure, which serves only to make the situation worse. How do we do this? We do it all the time, every day - during each one of the 14-16 hours a day we spend simply sitting or standing, and allowing the forces of gravity to push down on us.

The average adult head weighs between 11 and 13 pounds, and for all those 14 hours or more each day, it is squashing down on everything beneath it. All exercise movements, whether intended to help or not, will aggravate the damaged joint if they are done in a vertical plane, ie when sitting or standing. This means that strengthening and flexibility exercises designed to aid recovery may seem OK, but in fact they are fundamentally flawed if the spinal column is vertical during the activity.

THE ONLY SAFE AND EFFECTIVE BACK EXERCISES ARE THOSE CARRIED OUT WHEN THE BODY IS IN A HORIZONTAL PLANE.

Lying down is the most comfortable position for a person with backache. The vertebrae are 'suspended', with no postural stress, and so they can relax and the sufferer's pain is relieved. Lying down produces the least pressure on the spaces between the vertebrae, which is why the back actually lengthens during sleep. The natural curves of the back are exaggerated throughout the day, weighed down by fatigue, stresses and strains, but are straightened during sleep. Relieved of weight-bearing pressures, the discs are allowed to rehydrate, repair and recover.

There are many therapies available to the back sufferer, but the cheapest, simplest and most effective is that of stretching. Stretching the back is a subtle activity to be performed daily for life.

STARTING POSITION

Lie on your back with your knees bent and your feet together, soles flat on the floor, arms outstretched above the head.
Look up at the ceiling.

MOVEMENT

Slowly raise the pelvis to lift the hips off the floor. Keep your weight on heels and shoulders to form a bridge. Breathe normally. Now slowly move your pelvis a few inches over to the left, and then back to the right. Set up a gentle swaying motion. Keep the neck flat against the floor.

EFFECT

This is a very subtle mobilisation for the upper back which works out deep-seated muscle tension. Keeping the neck long and lengthened is an integral part of a healthy spine.

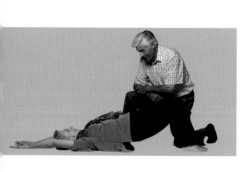

The benefits may take a little longer to be felt, but this method is gentler to the back and the effects are long-term. Stretching removes pain and restores function, dissolving the stiffness which started the discomfort.

The weekly routine which follows is designed specifically to counter poor posture, muscle spasm and restricted movements, and to allow the spine once again to function properly. For more than 10 years I myself suffered from a severe back condition. I studied ways to correct my own spinal curvature and carefully developed a repeating Five Day Exercise Routine.

Now I have good posture and have been pain-free since using this routine. In solving my own problems, I also discovered a way to give real hope to other back-pain sufferers.

My golden rule is this.

LIE DOWN TO DO BACK EXERCISES.

Doing exercises in the horizontal plane allows the spine to be stretched without the weight of the body exerting compression on any joints which are damaged or not functioning properly. The exercises in this book are safe, simple and ultra-friendly. No matter if you are an injured athlete in your twenties or a grandmother in your seventies, you too can safely and successfully do these exercises.

Horizontal stretching gently opens out and straightens that bent or hunched-over back, giving you a mobile and fully functioning spine. It is all unbelievably simple - so simple, it really works.

STARTING POSITION

Lying flat on your back, extend both arms above your head, legs stretched out.

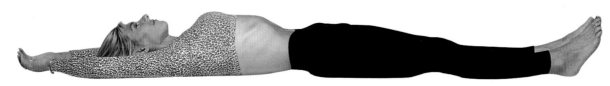

MOVEMENT

Taking the weight on the shoulders and the heels, lift your hips up off the floor to create a mini-arch. Look up at the ceiling. Breathe naturally. Gently sway the hips a few inches from side to side.

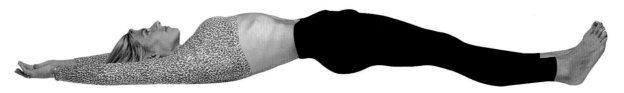

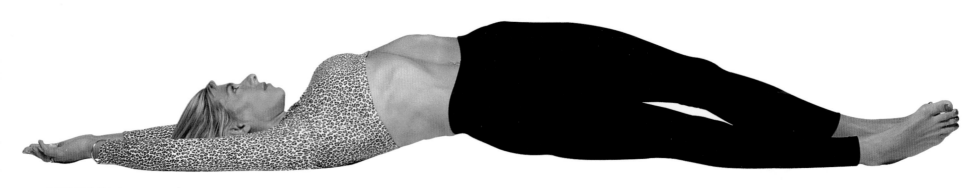

EFFECT

Feel the massage effect in the shoulders and upper back. You should feel your buttocks tighten and a stretch in the rib cage as well as a general lengthening effect along the whole of the spine. Tension and stiffness in the shoulder region are slowly released.

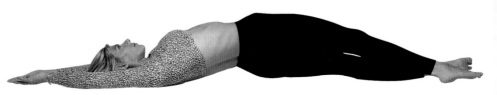

How to use this book

Flip and move – that's the way to read this book.

Flip over to Monday – Day One of your Five-Day Exercise program.

Now stand the book on the floor and flip over to the first exercise (Monday 1). Do the exercise and flip over to the next one (Monday 2). Complete the 7 exercises for Monday. Next day, work from Tuesday 1 through Tuesday 7.

Turn the book round and you will find Wednesday 1 on the other side. Now flip on through the daily exercises to Friday 7. When you have completed the Five-Day program - take a break, you deserve it! The following week, just turn the book round and start again at Monday 1.

Knee Lift: Right and Left Crucifix

STARTING POSITION
Lie flat on your back, legs straight, arms outstretched to make the shape of a crucifix.

MOVEMENT
Draw both knees slowly up towards the right hand, keeping the shoulders and the lower knee on the floor at all times. Keep your feet and knees together. Return to the starting position and repeat to the other side. Hold and perform five times on each side.

EFFECT
The effect is to stretch and lengthen the muscles of the lower back, removing stress and strain. Feel the twist in the lower back.

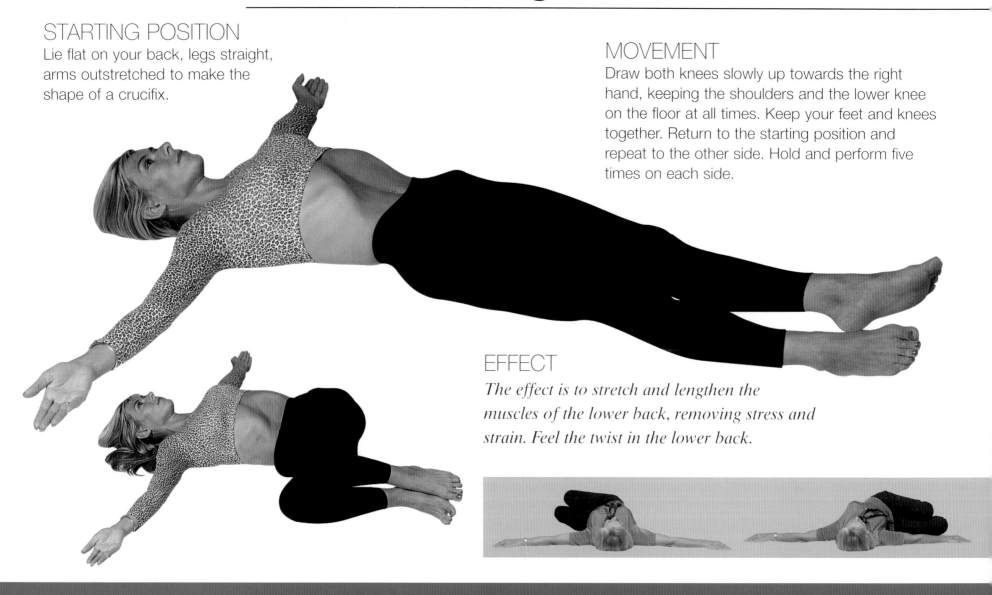

Shoulder Twist Sweep

STARTING POSITION

Lie flat on the floor on your back, legs apart and straight, arms out to the side at shoulder level, palms facing up.

MOVEMENT

Leaving your right arm flat on the floor, take your left hand across your chest and slide your left hand down your right arm, twisting at the shoulders. Look towards your hands and try to place the palms together. Try to keep your bottom in contact with the ground. From this position sweep the hands in a large circular movement above your head, keeping your hands in contact with the floor at all times. Continue the sweep, rolling across the top of your shoulders, until you reach the mirror-image position on the other side. Perform this sweeping motion six times.

EFFECT

This spinal twist releases muscle tension in the upper back and shoulder region. It will help you to regain the capacity to move in a way which may have been lost to you for years.

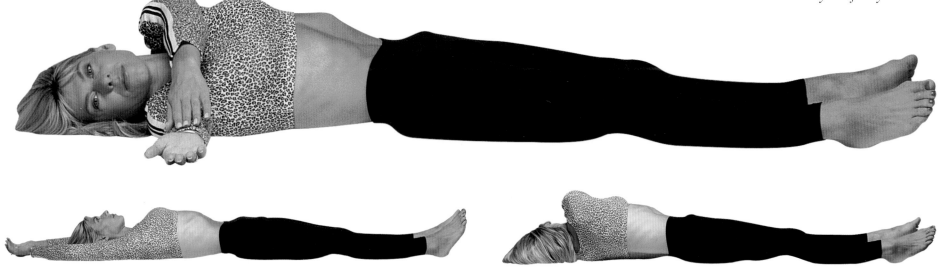

Five Days to a Healthy Back

The Back Coach's Daily Routine

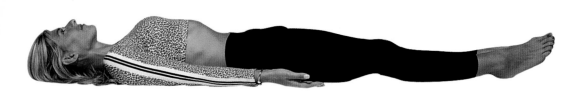

Total Back Relax

STARTING POSITION

Lie flat on your back, legs comfortably stretched out, arms resting by your side, the back of the hands resting on the floor. Breathe out through your nose.

MOVEMENT

Slowly breathe in through your nose, and at the same time sweep your arms around until the backs of the hands are resting on the floor directly over your head. At the height of the stretch, focus on stretching the hands away from the body and fully lengthening the spine. Hold for a moment, slowly breathe out through your nose and lower your arms to return to your starting position.
Perform five times.

EFFECT

You should feel a wave of relaxation go through your body. Moving like this prevents the vertebrae from sticking together, gently prising free discs which are squashed one on top of the other.

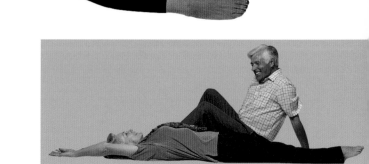

Introducing our team

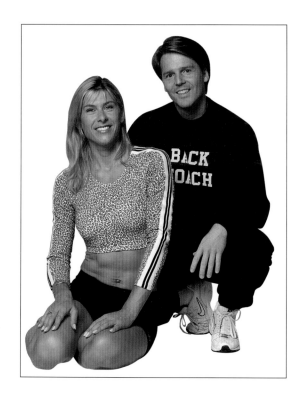

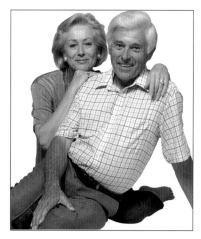

Sharron Davies is a former Olympic swimmer, Gold Medal athlete and now TV presenter.

Sharron started international swimming at the age of ten and competed for her country in three Olympics in three different decades, a career spanning some twenty years. After winning medals in every major championship she retired in the mid Nineties to pursue a new career in broadcasting. She has a young family and manages to combine motherhood with a full time profession, as well as still maintaining a high level of personal fitness. After a two year appearance on Gladiators, a very physical TV show, she sustained a knee injury which led to back problems that she now keeps under control with the use of these simple but effective back exercises.

Carole and Maurice are happily into the Third Age and they are doing just fine. They really enjoyed working through this new Five Day Exercise program. And, as you will see, they came through looking every bit as supple as Sharron.

Friday

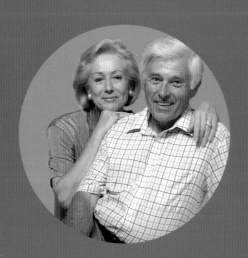

day 5

Total Back Relax

Shoulder Twist Sweep

Knee Lift: Right and Left Crucifix

Lying Flat Lift Hips - Rock

Swaying Bridge

Both Knees Press
against Chest - Rock

Cat on All-fours: Curl,
Stretch and Walk

Monday

day 1

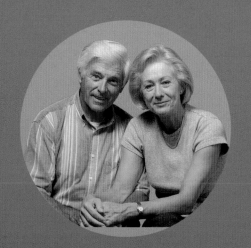

Walking on All-fours

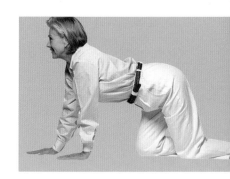

STARTING POSITION

On all-fours, with your weight evenly distributed between your hands and knees. Hands should be shoulder width apart, the knees slightly apart.

MOVEMENT

Move your left hand forward and at the same time move the right knee forward. Follow this immediately by moving the right hand and the left knee forward. It is possible to walk on your hands and knees in this fashion. Make five movements forward and five backward.

EFFECT

It is no coincidence that people suffering from back pain the world over revert to this position when pain strikes. Try it when you are feeling good and avoid discomfort later. The vertebrae are suspended with no postural stress, so where a joint is not functioning harmoniously with its neighbours it can take up its natural position without added stress and strains.

Back Lengthener

STARTING POSITION
Lie flat on your back, knees bent, feet flat on the floor.
Lightly hold your forearms, elbows raised in front of your chest.
Look straight up at the ceiling.

EFFECT
You will feel the stretch in your rib cage and along the full length of the spine. The spine will lengthen as you relax. This simple stretch helps to de-squash or decompress the spongy discs, prising them free and helping the spine to move and function as it was designed.

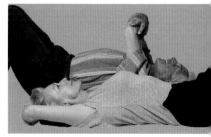

Relaxing in this way takes absolutely no effort.

MOVEMENT
Bring your arms back over your head until the forearms are resting on the floor.
Relax for a moment, then bring your arms forward over your head, through the starting position, to rest on your tummy. And relax.
Perform the whole sequence slowly five times.
Make all movements smooth, controlled and continuous. Breathe naturally at all times.

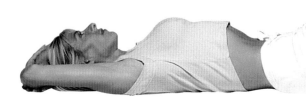

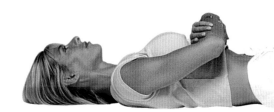

Cat on All-fours: Curl and Stretch

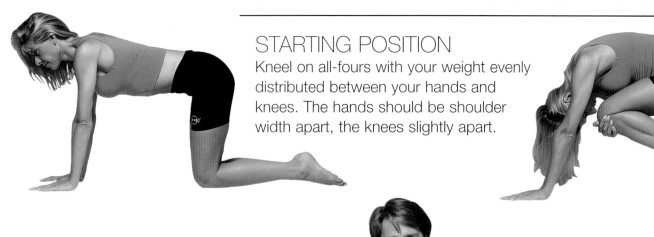

STARTING POSITION

Kneel on all-fours with your weight evenly distributed between your hands and knees. The hands should be shoulder width apart, the knees slightly apart.

MOVEMENT

Take hold of your left knee with your right hand. Curl your head towards your chest and pull the knee into the chest. Hold for a moment, then uncurl outwards, slowly extending the left leg until it is horizontal to the floor. At the same time extend the right hand horizontally out in front. This movement should be performed slowly and in a controlled manner.

Make sure to keep your back in a straight line. The hand, head and foot should be in a straight line and not arched. Return to the starting position and repeat with the opposite hand and knee. Perform the sequence five times on both sides. (If you find it too difficult to balance at first, keep both hands on the floor and move the leg only, until you have strengthened your back and have got accustomed to this movement.)

EFFECT

Try to feel the buttocks relax in the curled position, and tighten them in the uncurled straight body positions. This stretch ensures the discs are maintained in good health by allowing them to move freely.

Right and Left Knee Press against Chest

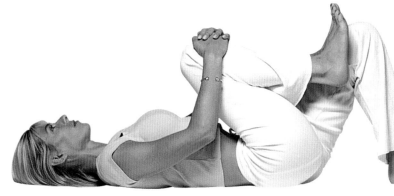

STARTING POSITION
Lie flat on your back, legs straight out and slightly apart.
Bend the left knee, keeping your foot flat on the floor.
Bring the right leg up and clasp the right knee with both hands. Look straight up at the ceiling.
Breathe naturally.

If it is difficult to raise the head, leave the head on the floor and hug the knee.

MOVEMENT
Breathe in, then slowly and gently pull the right knee toward your chest and at the same time raise your head as if to kiss your knee. Breathe out as you come up. Hold for a moment, then return to the starting position. And relax. Perform five times. Now do the same movement with the left leg. Perform five times.

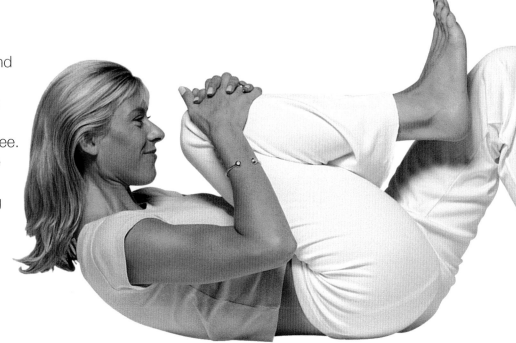

EFFECT
You will feel a tightness in the buttock region, and the lower lumbar will flatten against the floor. This stretch encourages our body to move in a dynamic, athletic way and helps to increase our range of movement types.

Reverse Abdominal/Lower Lumbar Strengtheners

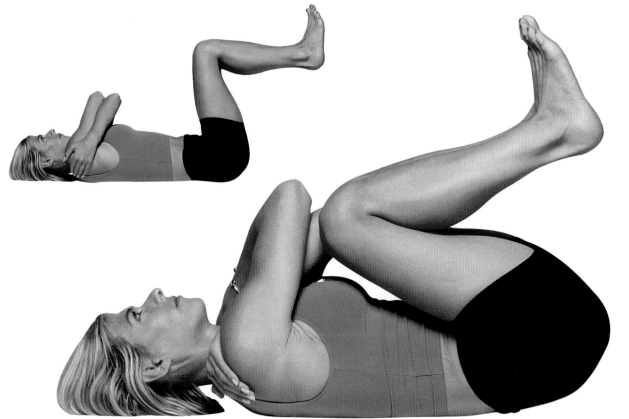

STARTING POSITION
Lie on your back, knees bent, the thighs perpendicular to the floor and the toes pointing up to the ceiling. Wrap your arms around you so your fingertips are touching your shoulder blades. Your elbows should be pointing up to the ceiling.

MOVEMENT
As you breathe out, rock the legs slightly toward your head. Lift the pelvis to round the lower lumbar. Repeat five times. Slowly lower the legs. And relax.

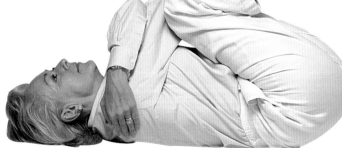

EFFECT
This is a subtle stretch of the lower lumbar, and the rocking motion massages the back. Strong stomach muscles are important not only because they make you look good, but because they are essential for keeping a pain-free back.

Lying Flat Stretch

STARTING POSITION

Lie flat on your back on the floor, your right arm outstretched over your head. The left arm is relaxed by your side. Stretch out your left leg and bend your right knee, keeping the sole of your foot flat on the floor.

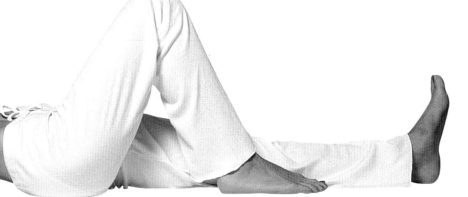

MOVEMENT

Now try to stretch the right arm and the left leg further away from the body. Stretch out, hold for a count of three and relax. Breathe naturally throughout. Do this movement five times.

Do the same stretch the other way round, with the left arm and right leg extended, and the right arm and left leg relaxed. Hold for a count of three and relax. Do this movement five times.

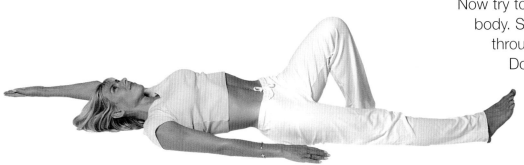

EFFECT

This movement creates a subtle rotation which you will feel around the pelvis. As you stretch away with arm and leg, try to develop the feeling that these limbs are lengthening.

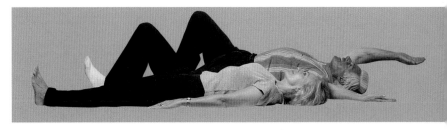

Never force or strain movements. Go as far as you comfortably can and relax.

Walking Bridge

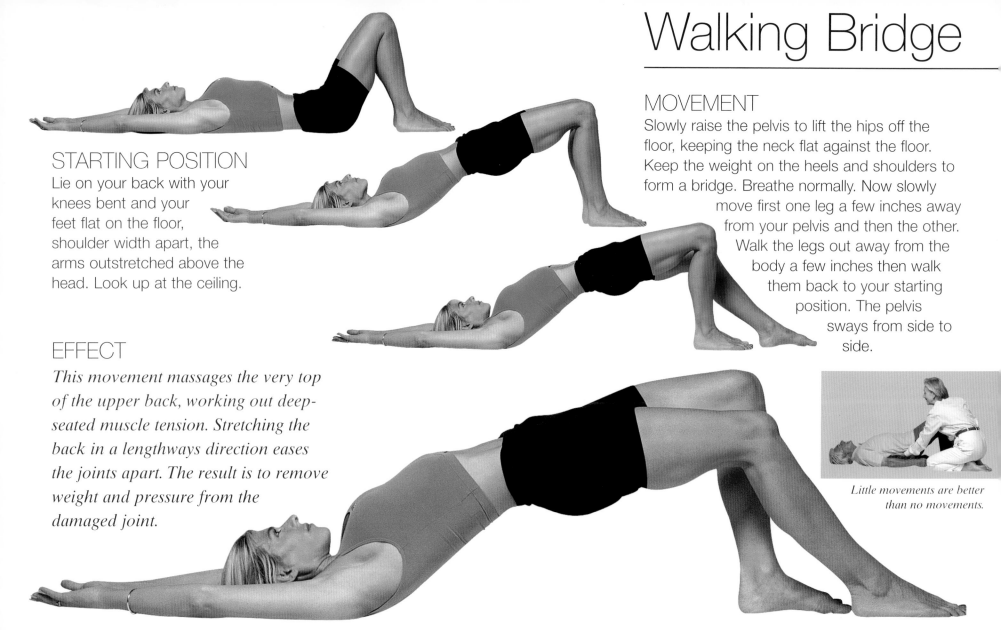

STARTING POSITION

Lie on your back with your knees bent and your feet flat on the floor, shoulder width apart, the arms outstretched above the head. Look up at the ceiling.

EFFECT

This movement massages the very top of the upper back, working out deep-seated muscle tension. Stretching the back in a lengthways direction eases the joints apart. The result is to remove weight and pressure from the damaged joint.

MOVEMENT

Slowly raise the pelvis to lift the hips off the floor, keeping the neck flat against the floor. Keep the weight on the heels and shoulders to form a bridge. Breathe normally. Now slowly move first one leg a few inches away from your pelvis and then the other. Walk the legs out away from the body a few inches then walk them back to your starting position. The pelvis sways from side to side.

Little movements are better than no movements.

Bridge

STARTING POSITION

Lie on your back with your knees bent and your feet slightly apart, flat on the floor, arms outstretched above your head. Look straight up at the ceiling. Breathe naturally.

EFFECT

You will feel a slight release in muscle tension as the floor applies pressure to those tight shoulder muscles.
Tuck the chin in to allow the neck to flatten. Feel the arms stretching away from the pelvis.

The beauty of these exercises is that they can be easily performed by anyone from superstar athletes to grandmothers.

MOVEMENT

Breathe in, then out as you slowly raise your pelvis to lift the hips off the floor. Keep your weight on the heels and shoulders to form a bridge. Hold for a moment, breathing naturally, and relax, then return to the starting position. Repeat five times.

Lying Flat Stretch with Pelvis Roll

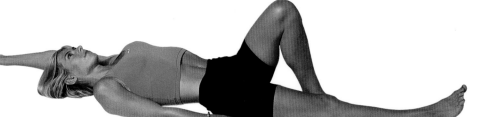

STARTING POSITION

Lie flat on your back on the floor, the left arm outstretched over the head, the right arm relaxed by your side. At the same time the right leg is stretched out and the left leg is bent, foot flat on the floor.

EFFECT

Feel a rocking motion around your pelvis. Rocking in this way gently loosens up the lower lumbar. Stretching in this way prevents the spine from sticking together, gently prising free discs which are squashed one on top of the other.

MOVEMENT

In this position you should aim to stretch the arm and leg further away from the body. Leading with the left knee, sway it six inches over the centreline of the body, and let it sway back to its starting position. Sway across for six movements. Change leg and repeat the movement on the other side.

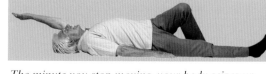

The minute you stop moving, your body seizes up. Keep the mobility and range of movement you have by moving every day.

Shoulder Twist

STARTING POSITION

Lie flat on your back on the floor, legs apart and straight, the arms out to the side at shoulder level, palms upwards.

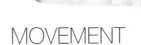

MOVEMENT

Leaving your right arm flat on the floor, bring your left hand across your chest and slide it down your right arm, twisting at the shoulders. Looking towards your hands, place the palms together. Try to keep your bottom in contact with the floor. Hold this position for a moment, then return to your starting position. Breathe naturally throughout.

Repeat this movement to the other side.

Perform five times on both sides.

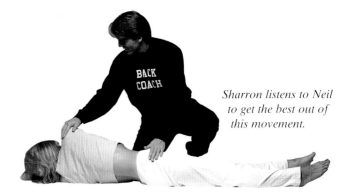

Sharron listens to Neil to get the best out of this movement.

EFFECT

This spinal twist releases muscle tension in the upper back and shoulder region, helping you to re-align your posture.

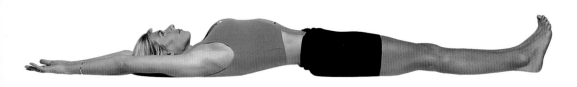

Lying Flat Lift Hips

STARTING POSITION

Lying flat on your back, extend both arms above your head, legs stretched out.

MOVEMENT

Taking the weight on the shoulders and the heels, lift your hips up off the floor to create a mini arch. Hold for a moment, looking up at the ceiling. Breathe naturally. Repeat five times.

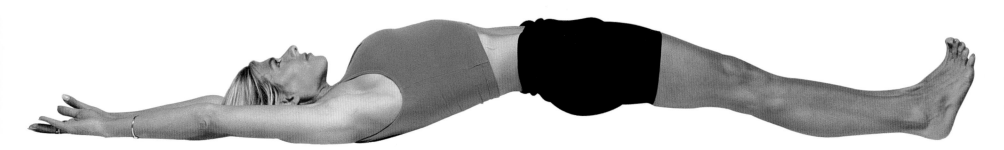

EFFECT

You should feel your buttocks tighten and a stretch in the rib cage as well as a general lengthening effect along the whole of the spine. Tension and stiffness in the shoulder region are slowly released.

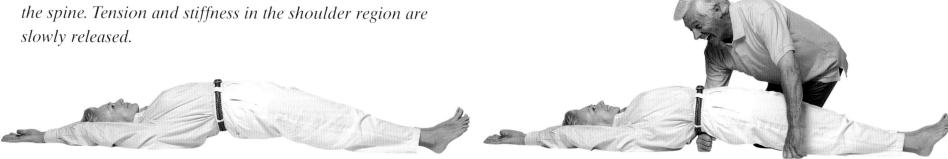

STARTING POSITION

Begin by kneeling, then lean forward and rest on your forearms in the all-fours position.

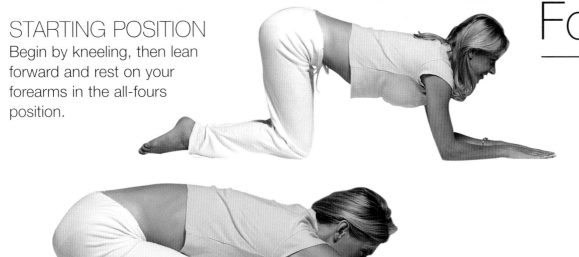

EFFECT

You should feel your head stretching away from your pelvis. Concentrate on lengthening the spine and drawing the head away from the pelvis. This movement helps the spine to become supple and strong.

MOVEMENT

Try to sit back on your heels, and at the same time straighten your arms out in front of you. Breathe naturally throughout.

Now bring the arms back to rest on the forearms, moving your upper body forward.

As you do so, slide the forearms forward and lower the pelvis slowly to the ground.

(You may need to adjust your forearms to be in line with your head as you move forward.)

Perform the complete movement five times in a flowing continuous sequence.

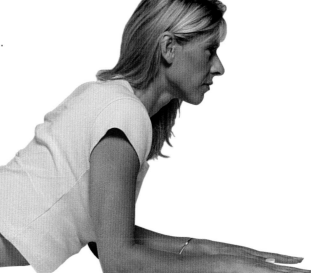

STARTING POSITION

Lie flat on your back, knees bent, feet flat on the floor. Hold the forearms lightly interlocked, resting on the floor above your head.

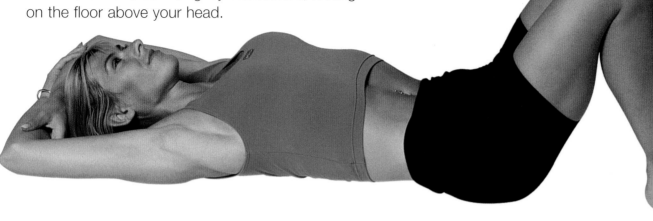

EFFECT

Lengthways stretching helps to free each vertebra from impacting with the one below. By encouraging this stretch we help to move the impacted vertebra off the bottom one, thus taking the pressure off the damaged area.

MOVEMENT

Backwalking is completed by circling the arms in a sweeping motion. Move the arms first to the left, sweeping down over the tummy and on up the right-hand side. Sweep the arms round in a circular fashion, making large circles with the inter-locked forearms. Circle 5 times in one direction. Repeat the process with the forearms moving in the opposite direction. Again circle 5 times.

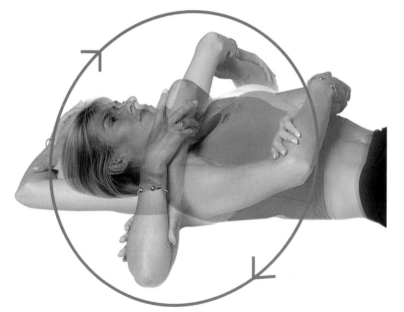

If you only do one exercise before you go to bed each night, it should be this one.

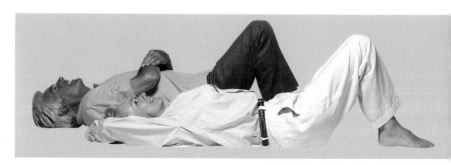

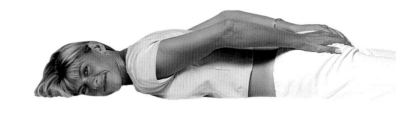

STARTING POSITION

Lie face down flat on the floor, the head turned to the left, and with the palms of the hands resting on the buttocks. Make sure your legs are together and firmly on the floor.

MOVEMENT

Slide the hands down the backs of the thighs. At the same time, raise the head slowly and, keeping it turned to the left, bring your shoulders upward and off the floor.

Hold for a moment, then return slowly and in a controlled manner to your starting position. Relax. It is important to turn the head to one side to prevent the neck from hyper-extending and being pulled back too far. Perform the movement five times with the head facing to the left, and then repeat five times with the head to the right.

EFFECT

As you bring your body up and turn your head sideways, you are trying to move the head out and away from the pelvis. This helps to stretch the spine in a lengthways direction.

This is an excellent way to strengthen those all important back muscles. Tense the muscles of the back and buttocks as you draw the head up.

Thursday

day 4

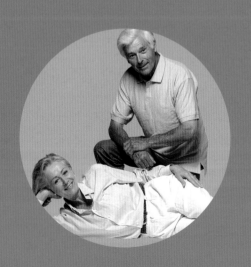

Backwalking

Lying Flat Lift Hips

Lying Flat Stretch with Pelvis Roll

Walking Bridge

Reverse Abdominal/ Lower Lumbar Strengtheners

Cat on All-fours: Curl and Stretch

Walking on All-fours

Tuesday

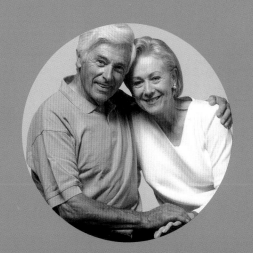

day 2

Straight Stretch Hold

Both Knees Press against Chest

Face up Chest Lift

Rock and Wrap

Face down Chest Raise

Forearm Walk

Curled Ball

STARTING POSITION

Kneeling on all-fours, place your right knee ahead of your left knee, splitting the legs to create a more stable base. Both your hands are shoulder width apart.

EFFECT

This stretch reverses our tendency as a sedentary being to bend and flex in monotonous unhelpful ways. It restores movement in the joints, stopping them from 'drying out' and allowing them to regain elasticity.

MOVEMENT

From this position keep your right hand on the floor, and sweep your left hand underneath your body to touch the right shoulder blade. Now sweep this left hand back under the body and reach for the ceiling, opening out the chest and twisting the spine to the left. Try to look up at the ceiling. Hold for a moment at the top and relax. Repeat five times. Return to the starting position. Do the exercise to the other side, sweeping with the right arm. Repeat five times.

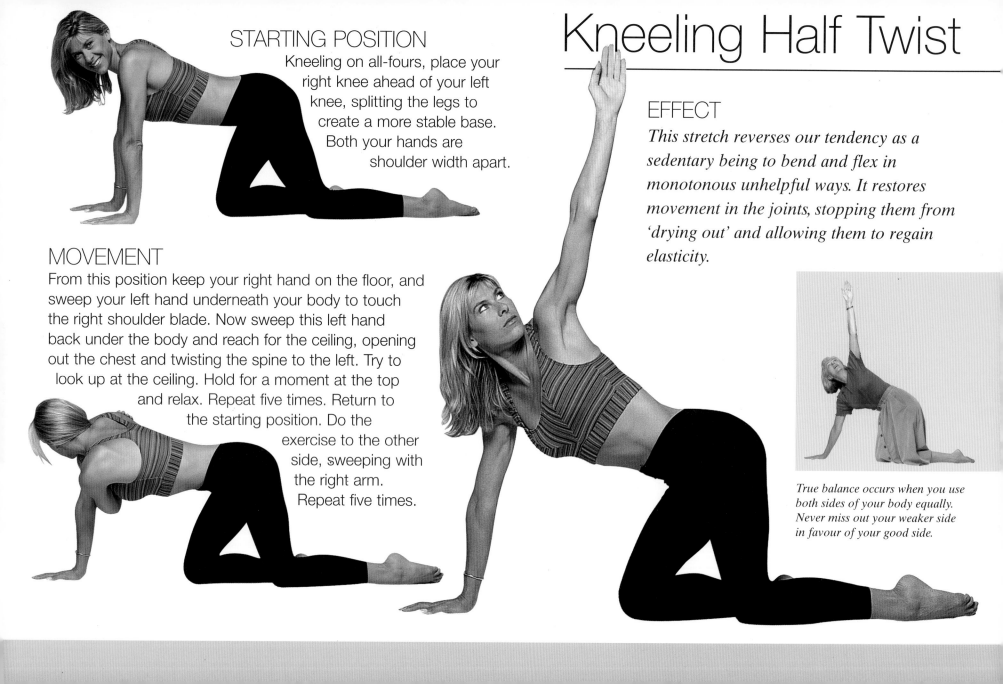

True balance occurs when you use both sides of your body equally. Never miss out your weaker side in favour of your good side.

STARTING POSITION

Lie flat on your back, knees bent, feet flat on the floor, both arms stretched straight above the head, the backs of the hands touching.

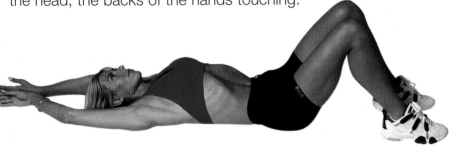

Straight Stretch Hold

MOVEMENT

Cross one hand over the other until the palms are facing and touching each other. Squeeze the hands together and stretch away from the body. Hold for 10 seconds. Repeat with the other hand crossing over. Hold for 10 seconds. Perform the whole sequence five times on both sides.

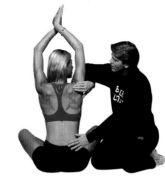

Stretch, squeeze and relax. This tones and strengthens as well as stretches.

EFFECT

As you squeeze, feel the tension in the back of the shoulders. Try to create the feeling of the arms moving away from the pelvis to encourage the spine to lengthen. Not allowing it to become overly compressed is the best gift you can give your spine.

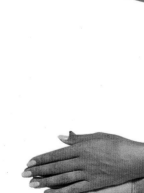

Abdominal Stomach Strengtheners

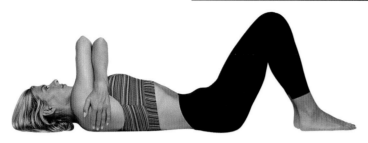

STARTING POSITION

Lie on your back, knees bent, feet flat on the floor. Wrap your arms around you so your fingertips are touching your shoulder blades. Your elbows should be pointing up to the ceiling. Hold and squeeze for a moment.

MOVEMENT

Raise your head slightly and curl the upper part of the back forward. Breathe out, tightening the stomach muscles at the same time. Lower slowly. And relax. Repeat five times.

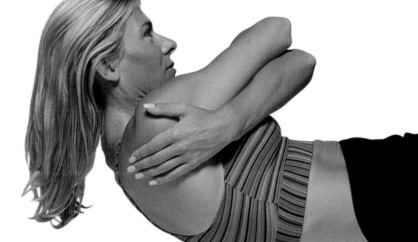

EFFECT

Strong stomach muscles are essential for a pain-free back. By curling the spine in this manner it is possible to tense and shorten the stomach muscles, giving them an intense workout.

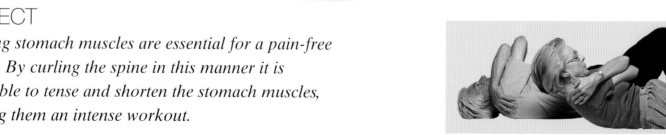

Both Knees Press against Chest

STARTING POSITION
Lie on your back, bend both knees toward the chest and clasp both knees with both hands. And relax.

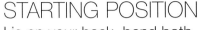

MOVEMENT
Gently pull in both knees towards the chest and at the same time raise the head as though to kiss the knees. Breathe out as you move. Hold for a moment, return to the starting position and repeat five times.

If it is too hard at first to lift your head, just curl from the lower lumbar, leaving the head resting on the floor.

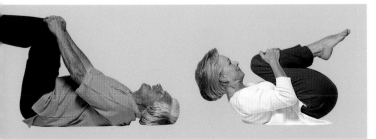

EFFECT
Feel the stretch in the lower back and buttocks. Regain the feeling of a supple and agile spine. Stretching in this way removes stiffness and restores function.

Side Bends in Lying Position

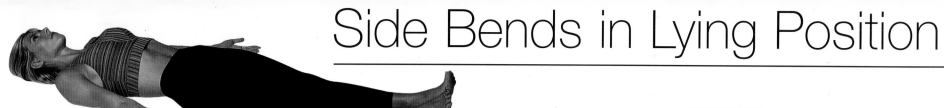

EFFECT

Doing this stretch in the horizontal plane allows the spine to stretch without the weight of the body exerting a compressing element on the joints. It helps to promote correct posture and ensures that all other joints in the spine are in their optimum working positions.

STARTING POSITION

Lie flat on your back in a relaxed position, legs straight out and arms by your side, palms upward.

MOVEMENT

Raise your chin slightly by lifting your head and at the same time slide your right hand down the side of your right leg. Return to the starting position. Do the same on the left side. Perform the sequence five times.

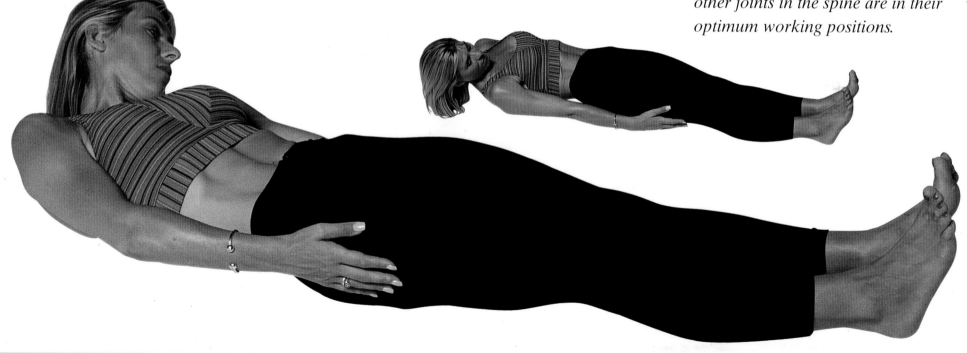

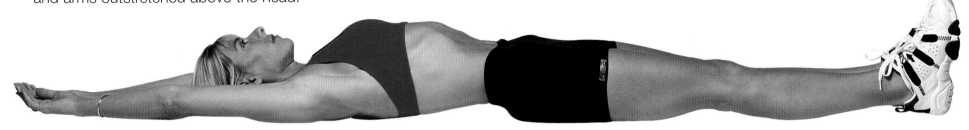

STARTING POSITION

Lie flat on the floor on your back, legs straight and arms outstretched above the head.

MOVEMENT

Keeping the heels, bottom and head on the floor, raise the chest allowing the shoulders to come away from the floor. Hold for a moment. Lower and relax. Repeat the movement five times.

Sharron's flexibility is amazing, as you can imagine. Do not get discouraged if your movement is more restricted when starting. Practice makes perfect.

EFFECT

This stretch is designed to counter poor posture, muscle spasm and restricted movement, allowing the spine once again to function properly. This builds up strength in the neck which is sadly lacking for most of us.

STARTING POSITION

Lie flat on your back, knees bent, feet flat on the floor and together. Both arms outstretched above the head, the backs of the hands touching.

MOVEMENT

Cross one hand over the other until the palms are facing and touching each other. Squeeze the hands together and stretch away from the body. With just the slightest movement rock the hips from side to side, the knees gently swaying six inches to either side. Sway for six movements. Repeat with the other hand crossing over.

Stiffness and restricted movement creep up on us over many years. Be patient with yourself as you gradually loosen up over the coming weeks and months.

EFFECT

This gentle movement frees up the lower back. As the back muscles regain their natural muscle tone, the back straightens and youthful posture returns. Muscles loosen and lengthen, creating a relaxed back free from fatigue.

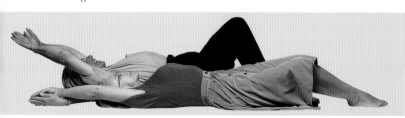

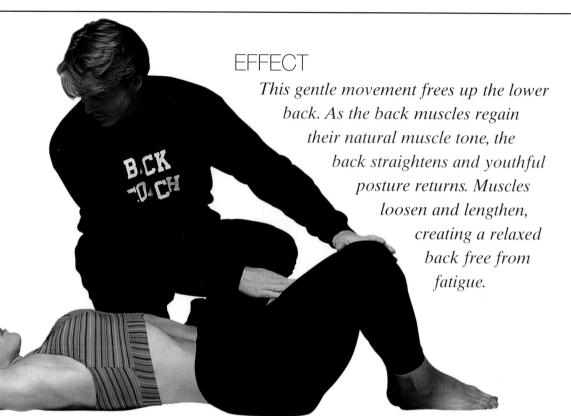

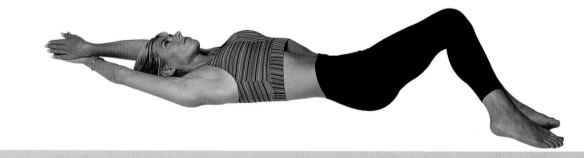

STARTING POSITION

Lie flat on your back, knees bent, feet flat on the floor. Wrap your arms around you so your fingertips are touching your shoulder blades. The elbows should be pointing up to the ceiling. Hold and squeeze for a moment.

EFFECT

You should feel a gentle massaging effect across the upper back and shoulders. This stretch promotes a healthy relaxed back, posturally aligned and moving as nature intended.

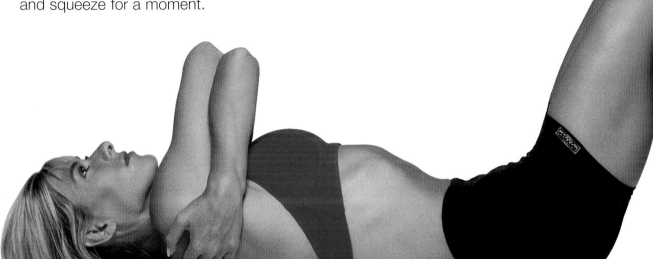

MOVEMENT

Keeping your feet still and your legs and pelvis stationary, rock/sway your elbows from side to side. Keep looking up to the ceiling.

Just squeezing creates a fantastic release in deep-seated muscle tension.

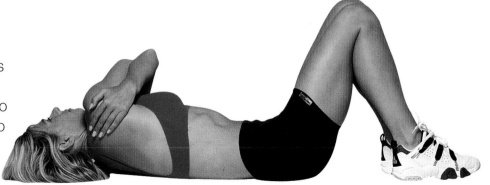

Isometric Neck Press

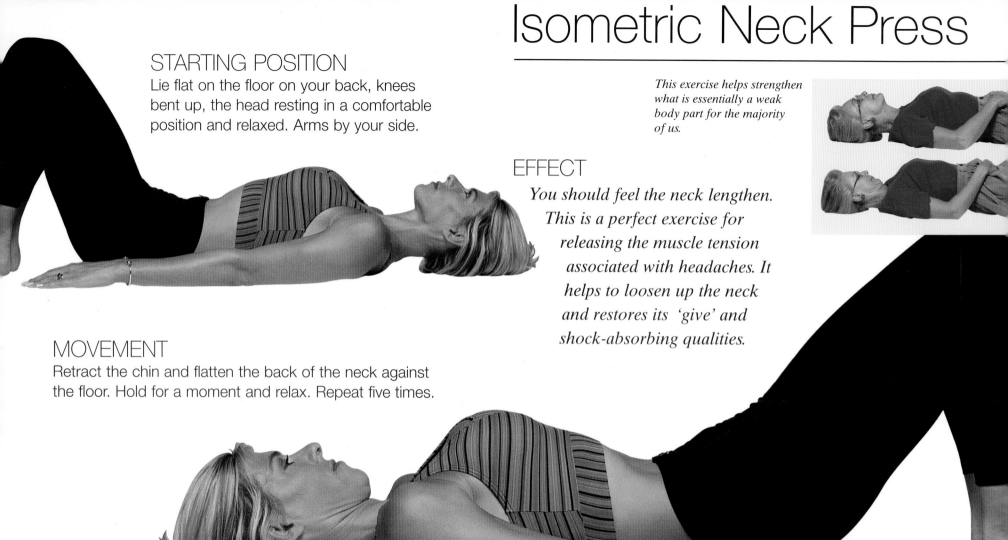

STARTING POSITION

Lie flat on the floor on your back, knees bent up, the head resting in a comfortable position and relaxed. Arms by your side.

This exercise helps strengthen what is essentially a weak body part for the majority of us.

EFFECT

You should feel the neck lengthen. This is a perfect exercise for releasing the muscle tension associated with headaches. It helps to loosen up the neck and restores its 'give' and shock-absorbing qualities.

MOVEMENT

Retract the chin and flatten the back of the neck against the floor. Hold for a moment and relax. Repeat five times.

Face down Chest Raise

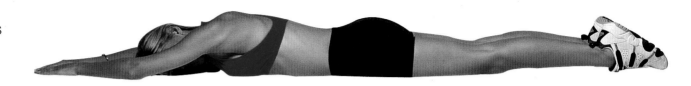

STARTING POSITION

Lie face down flat on the floor, the legs together, arms outstretched above the head. Relax and breathe naturally.

MOVEMENT

Keeping the hands where they are, raise the head and chest only. Turn the head to one side. Hold at the top of the stretch. Return to the starting position. Repeat five times on both sides.

Olympic superstar or not, this routine is simplicity itself.

EFFECT

As you draw the head up and out, you should feel a stretch in the upper back. This movement helps to straighten out that bent/hunched back.

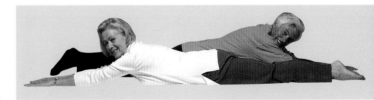

These stretches are for the home, you don't have to go to the gym to benefit. In your everyday clothes and on your lounge floor...that's just fine.

Lower Lumbar Press against Floor

STARTING POSITION

Lie flat on your back, bend both knees up, the feet flat on the floor. Wrap your arms around you with the fingertips on the shoulders. Feel the natural curve in your lower lumbar. Look straight up at the ceiling.

MOVEMENT

As you breathe out, flatten your lower lumbar against the floor and at the same time tighten up your tummy muscles. Hold for a moment and repeat five times.

EFFECT

The lower lumbar takes the brunt of the overload caused by sitting and poor postural positions. This stretch removes that load from the spine and brings relief to the lower back region.

Forearm Walk

STARTING POSITION
Lie flat on the floor, face down, then raise the head and shoulders to rest on your forearms.

EFFECT
This is one of the best ways to stretch the spine. Stretching lengthways eases the joints away from each other, keeping things open and functioning as they were designed.

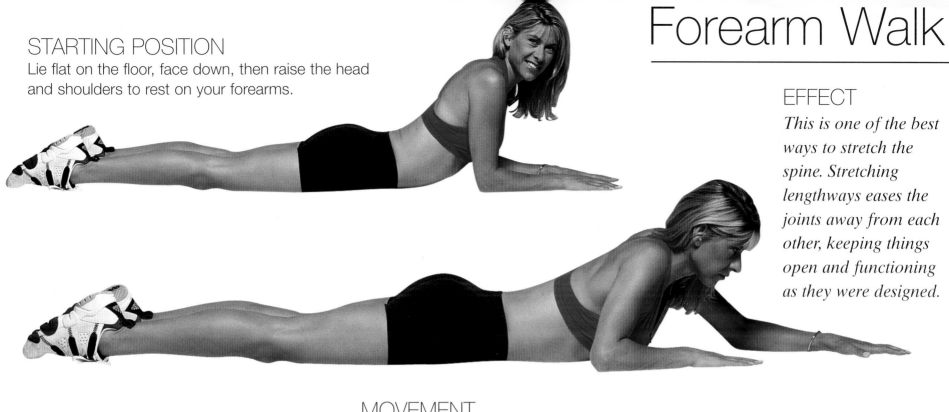

MOVEMENT
From this position inch forward one forearm after the other, drawing yourself forward as if crawling on your forearms. Relax the legs. The hips rotate from side to side.

Encourage the traction effect by allowing the legs to drag 'dead weight' behind as you crawl forward.

STARTING POSITION

Lie flat on your back, bend both knees up, feet flat on the floor. Lightly hold your forearms, elbows raised in front of your chest. Look up at the ceiling.

Back Loosener

EFFECT

You should feel the dead weight of the arms subtly stretch the back and shoulders. In this position the weight has been taken off the intervertebral spaces. Relieved of pressure, the discs can rehydrate, repair and recover. As the back loosens up, it eventually stretches its way to its natural pain-free position.

Whether it is listening to your favourite CD or to the evening news, it's easy to find a few minutes each day to do these stretches.

MOVEMENT

Sway the arms over to the right until the right elbow and the back of the right upper arm are resting gently on the floor. And relax. Now sway the arms in the other direction. Move smoothly back through the starting position, all the way until the left upper arm and elbow are resting on the floor. And relax. Breathe naturally while performing all movements. Repeat this sequence five times.

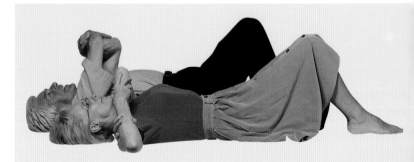

STARTING POSITION

Kneeling down, sit on your heels. Curl forward to place your forehead as close to the floor near your knees as you can, arms outstretched in front, palms flat on the floor.

Curled Ball

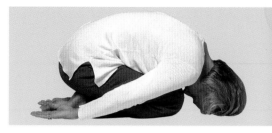

Each time you breathe out feel yourself sink further into deep relaxation.

MOVEMENT

As you become more relaxed, take a deep breath, breathe out and sweep the arms around until the backs of the hands are on the floor near your heels. And relax. Remain in this position for several minutes.

EFFECT

This stretch de-squashes the spine. As you relax further into this stretch, feel the spine lengthen from the pelvis to the head. The tightness in the lower back is released.

Wednesday

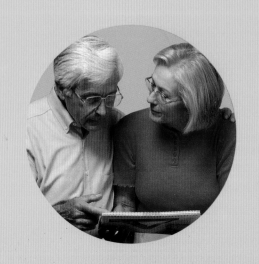

day 3